THE SWEET POTATO SOLUTION

A Delicious Path to Health and Wellness

Ray Y. Manuel

ABOUT THE AUTHOR

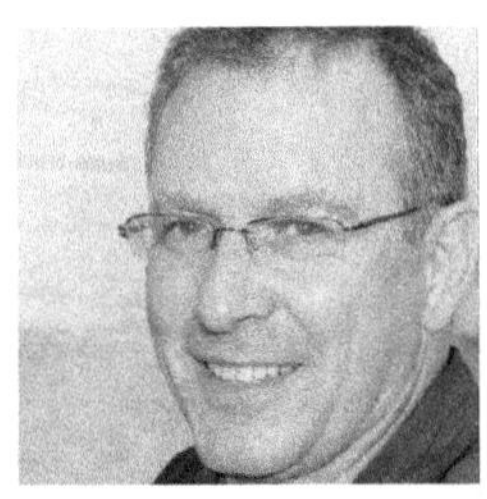

Ray Y. Manuel, M.D. is a well-regarded physician from the United States who has been practicing for over 20 years. Throughout his long career, Dr. Manuel has been known for his commitment to patient care and his fervent support of health and well-being in the US. His knowledge and skills are diverse, allowing him to be a well-rounded and informed doctor.

Dr. Manuel is a passionate health advocate who works to inform the public about the value of preventative care and nutrition in addition to his medical practice. As an Author, Dr. Manuel offers readers a thorough guide for improved health by fusing his medical knowledge with his love of living a healthy lifestyle.

In his medical practice, Dr. Manuel focuses on the relationship between nutrition and general health, and he aims to provide people with the knowledge and skills they need to make decisions that will benefit their long-term health. He is regarded as a prominent figure in the field of health advocacy since his work continues to motivate many people to lead healthier lifestyles.

TABLE OF CONTENTS

CHAPTER 1
INTRODUCTION TO SWEET POTATOES

The dicotyledonous sweet potato (Ipomoea batatas) is a member of the Convolvulaceae family, which also includes bindweed and morning glory. Root vegetables are made from big, starchy, sweet-tasting tuberous roots. On occasion, the young leaves and shoots are used as greens. Sweet potato cultivars have been bred to produce tubers with different colored meat and skin. Both sweet potatoes and common potatoes (Solanum tuberosum) belong to the same order, Solanales, and are only tangentially related. Though the species is even more distant from the actual yams, which are monocots in the order Dioscoreales, darker sweet potatoes are nonetheless known as "yams" in some parts of North America.

Native to what is now Ecuador, the sweet potato originated in the tropical regions of South America. I. batatas is the only important crop plant of the roughly 50 genera and more than 1,000 species of the Convolvulaceae family; the others are poisonous, though some are used locally (e.g., I. aquatica "kangkong" as a green vegetable). The sweet potato belongs to the genus Ipomoea, which also includes a few garden flowers known as morning gloryries, though I. batatas are not commonly included in that term. In horticulture, certain varieties of I. batatas are utilized as decorative plants and cultivated under the name tuberous morning glory. In North America, sweet potatoes are sometimes referred to as yams. There, when soft types were initially planted for commercial purposes, it was necessary to distinguish between the two. Because the soft' sweet potatoes resembled the unrelated yams in Africa, enslaved Africans had already begun calling them 'yams'.So, to differentiate soft sweet potatoes from 'firm' ones, they were called 'yams'.

Taxonomy

The sweet potato comes from what is now Ecuador in South America. Either Central America or South America is where sweet potatoes were first domesticated. Domesticated sweet potatoes were first domesticated at least 5,000 years ago in Central America; I. batatas may have originated between the mouth of the Orinoco River in Venezuela and the Yucatán Peninsula of Mexico. By 2500 BCE, the cultigen had most likely been transported by the locals to South America and the Caribbean.

The closest wild relative of the sweet potato is I. trifida, a diploid that was created by a second complete genome duplication event after an initial cross between a tetraploid and another diploid parent. The earliest known sweet potato remains, as determined by radiocarbon dating, were found in caves in the south-central region of Peru, in the Chilca Canyon. These bones offer an age of 8080 ± 170 BC.

Diets low in carbs are a common strategy for calorie restriction and weight loss. Despite their carbohydrate content, sweet potatoes still have nutrients to offer and can be a valuable addition to your diet.

Carbohydrates: An Overview
Four categories of carbohydrates exist:

- Basic natural substances like fructose in fruit or lactose in milk
- Basic refinement, like white sugar
- Complex natural foods like whole grains
- Legumes sophisticated refinement, like white flour

Add-ins like soda, candies, and cookies are made with refined carbs. They may have a detrimental effect on your blood sugar. When cutting back on carbohydrates, these are the ones you should steer clear of the most.

You consume fewer carbohydrates each day when you adhere to a low-carb diet. Rather, you consume more "healthy" fat and protein. Cutting back on carbohydrates causes your body to burn fat for energy rather than store it.

Reducing carbohydrates is typically done to lose weight. However, some low-carb diets have also been shown to reduce the incidence of type 2 diabetes and other disorders affecting how your body burns fuel.

The kinds of low-carb diets differ in what they permit. Some allow you to eat a couple of servings of veggies, whole grains, and fruit. Sweet potatoes have a role in these diets.

The Essentials of Sweet Potatoes
You could believe that sweet potatoes are simply a type of white potato. However, common potatoes are nightshade family members and are considered tubers. Sweet potatoes are a type of edible root that is related to morning glory.

Compared to white potatoes, sweet potatoes offer greater nutritional value. People tend not to consume sweet potatoes as much as they may with white potatoes, even though sweet potato fries are a popular dish.

Carbohydrates are abundant in sweet potatoes. A 5-inch sweet potato contains roughly 26 grams of carbs. One sweet potato contains half of the total calories from carbohydrates that you may be permitted to consume on a low-carb diet.

However, that is still less than the 35 grams on average found in a white potato. That's less than those fries with sweet potatoes as well. Their preparation increases their carbohydrate load to around 34 grams.

Sweet potatoes that are simply prepared can be included in low-carb diets that permit vegetables in moderation.

Sugar Potato Nutrient Content

Sweet potatoes have white, cream, orange, and purple flesh with a bronze skin tone. They are naturally sweet and nutrient-rich, including:

- Beta-carotene, a kind of vitamin A
- B6 vitamin
- Vitamin C
- Potassium
- Fiber

While purple sweet potatoes include a wealth of other antioxidants, orange sweet potatoes are high in vitamin A. These aid in shielding your body against waste products produced by your cells, known as free radicals. Some sources of free radicals include:

- Infection
- smoke from cigarettes
- Air contamination
- Sunlight

In addition, fiber from sweet potatoes is a complex carbohydrate that slows down both soluble and insoluble digestion. Fiber gives your stool moisture, which facilitates its easy passage through and elimination from your digestive system. Fiber can assist lower high blood sugar and cholesterol levels in addition to reducing your chance of intestinal issues.

How to Prepare Sweet Potatoes
Sweet potatoes should be kept dry and cold. To maximize the nutrients in them, it is advisable to use them within a week.
Scrub the sweet potato's skin clean before cooking, but don't remove it. The skin is a great source of fiber and is healthy.

They can be baked or sliced. They take eight to ten minutes to cook in the microwave, flipping them over halfway through. Alternatively, chop the potatoes into 1-inch pieces and cook them for 15 to 20 minutes at a rolling boil. Mashing cooked sweet potatoes is another option.

Sweet potatoes can be chopped and boiled and used in soups or salads if you wish to eat less of them to reduce your intake of carbohydrates. For a quick supper, you may also cut a cooked sweet potato in half and top it with a protein and maybe another low-carb ingredient.

Lowering your carbohydrate intake over time may cause you to lose some significant nutritional intake. Making the most of the carbohydrates you eat is what you should aim for. So remember that sweet potatoes are very nutritious.

See your doctor about vitamins and other supplements if you're still not getting enough nutrition from your diet.

CHAPTER 2
HEALTH BENEFITS OF SWEET POTATOES

Sweet potatoes are high in nutrients, with each serving containing notable levels of manganese, vitamin C, and vitamin A. In addition to their anticancer properties, they might boost immunity and offer other health benefits.

Sweet potatoes are starchy, sweet root vegetables that are cultivated all over the world.

They are abundant in vitamins, minerals, antioxidants, and fiber and come in a range of sizes and hues, such as orange, white, and purple.

Not to mention, they are simple to incorporate into your diet and offer a host of health advantages.

These are 6 unexpected advantages of sweet potatoes for your health.

1. Extremely nourishing

Sweet potatoes are a fantastic source of vitamins, minerals, and fiber.

200 grams (g) or one cup of cooked sweet potatoes with skins provide

- 180 calories, 41 grams of carbs
- 4 g of protein
- 0.3 g of fat
- 6.6 g of fiber
- 213% of the Daily Value (DV) for vitamin A
- Vit C: 44% of the Daily Value
- 43% of the DV is manganese.
- 36% of the DV is copper.
- (35% of the DV) for pantothenic acid
- B6: 34 percent of the daily value
- 20% of the DV is potassium.
- 19% of the DV for niacin

Furthermore, sweet potatoes are a great source of antioxidants that shield your body from free radicals, particularly the orange and purple types.

Unstable chemicals known as free radicals can damage DNA and cause inflammation.

Chronic diseases such as cancer, heart disease, and aging have all been related to damage caused by free radicals. Eating foods high in antioxidants is therefore beneficial to your health.

2. Encourage digestive wellness

Sweet potatoes' fiber and antioxidants may be good for your intestines.

There are two kinds of fiber in sweet potatoes: soluble and insoluble.

Both types are indigestible to your body. As a result, fiber remains in your digestive system and offers several health advantages relating to your gut.

Viscous fibers, a subtype of soluble fiber, can absorb water and soften stools. Conversely, non-viscous, insoluble fibers do not take in water and become more substantial.

The bacteria in your colon can ferment some soluble and insoluble fibers, producing substances known as short-chain fatty acids that support and maintain the health of the cells lining your intestines.

Diets high in fiber, including 20–33 g of fiber daily, have been associated with a decreased risk of colon cancer as well as more frequent bowel movements.

Sweet potatoes' antioxidants might also provide advantages for the digestive system.

Antioxidants in purple sweet potatoes have been shown in test-tube research to support the establishment of beneficial gut flora, such as several species of Lactobacillus and Bifidobacterium.

Increases in certain kinds of bacteria in the intestines are linked to improved gut health and a decreased incidence of diseases including infectious diarrhea and irritable bowel syndrome (IBS).

3. Might be able to combat cancer

A variety of antioxidants found in sweet potatoes may help prevent some malignancies.

In vitro experiments have demonstrated that anthocyanins, a class of antioxidants present in purple sweet potatoes, can inhibit the growth of specific cancer cell types, including bladder, colon, stomach, and breast cancers.

In a similar vein, rats given diets high in purple sweet potatoes had reduced incidence of colon cancer in its early stages, indicating that the potato's anthocyanins may offer some protection. Sweet potato peel extracts have also been shown to have anti-cancer properties in studies conducted on animals and in test tubes.

Studies on humans have not yet examined these impacts, though.

4. Encourage good eye health

The antioxidant known as beta carotene, which gives sweet potatoes their vivid orange hue, is abundant in these vegetables.

The daily requirement of beta carotene for the average adult is more than doubled by just one cup (200 g) of roasted orange sweet potatoes with skin.

Beta carotene is converted by your body into vitamin A, which is then used to make light-sensitive receptors in your eyes.

Severe vitamin A deficiency can cause xerophthalmia, a unique kind of blindness that is a concern in impoverished nations. Consuming foods high in beta-carotene, such as sweet potatoes with orange flesh, may help stave off this illness.

Additionally, purple sweet potatoes appear to aid vision.

Their ability to shield eye cells from harm has been demonstrated in earlier test-tube investigations, and this may have important implications for overall eye health.

5. Could improve mental performance

Purple sweet potatoes have been shown to enhance brain function.

According to animal research, the anthocyanins in purple sweet potatoes may lessen inflammation and shield the brain from damage caused by free radicals.

According to a different study, giving mice supplements enriched with anthocyanin-rich sweet potato extract may lower inflammatory indicators and enhance their spatial working memory. This could be because the extract has antioxidant qualities.

In general, diets high in fruits, vegetables, and antioxidants are linked to a 13% decreased risk of mental decline and dementia, yet no research has been done to evaluate these effects in humans.

6. Could bolster your defenses against illness

Sweet potatoes with orange flesh are among the best natural providers of beta carotene, a plant-based substance that your body uses to make vitamin A.

A robust immune system depends on vitamin A, and low blood levels of the vitamin have been connected to weakened immunity.

It's also essential for keeping mucous membranes in good condition, particularly the lining of your stomach.

Your body is exposed to numerous microorganisms that have the potential to cause disease in the gut. Consequently, a strong immune system depends in large part on a healthy gut.

Research indicates that a shortage in vitamin A worsens gut inflammation and impairs your immune system's capacity to react appropriately to possible dangers.

Although research on the potential effects of sweet potatoes in particular on immunity has not been done, eating them frequently can help avoid vitamin A deficiency.

Ways to include them in your diet

Including sweet potatoes in your diet is easy.

They can be baked, boiled, roasted, steamed, or pan-cooked, and eaten with or without the skin.

They can be used in both savory and sweet recipes because of their inherent sweetness, which goes well with a wide variety of seasonings.

Here are a few well-liked ways to eat sweet potatoes:

- Sweet potato chips are cooked after being peeled and thinly sliced.
- Peel, cut, and bake sweet potato fries into wedges or matchsticks.
- Sweet potato toast: Thinly slice, toast, and top with avocado or nut butter, if desired.

- Sweet potatoes are boiled, peeled, then mashed with salt and milk.
- Sweet potatoes baked whole: Baked till fork-tender in the oven.
- Peel, chop, and sauté sweet potatoes in a pan with onions and peppers.
- Cut sweet potatoes into spirals, then sauté and coat with sauce.
- Sweet potato puree provides moisture to baked foods without adding fat.

Since beta carotene is a fat-soluble nutrient, cooking sweet potatoes with a small amount of fat, such as avocado, coconut oil, or olive oil, can aid increase the absorption of this nutrient.

Some previous research has suggested that heating sweet potatoes somewhat lowers their beta-carotene concentration, but they still contain at least 70% of this mineral and are still regarded as a great source.

CHAPTER 3
PREPARATION AND RECIPES

You don't need to search any further for delicious and simple sweet potato recipes. Sweet potatoes are more than just an orange substitute for regular potatoes with white flesh. These root veggies are so distinctive and adaptable that they have their category of recipes, such as pies and bread, that you would never consider preparing with white potatoes.

Sweet potatoes are often thought of as delectable Thanksgiving side dishes, but they can also be cooked quickly enough to serve on a weeknight dinner plate. This makes them ideal for winter nights when you're yearning for something warm and cozy.

Each recipe, which includes appetizers, side dishes, snacks, and desserts, was created to showcase the qualities of the sweet potato, such as its inherent sweetness, velvety flesh, and adaptability. Regardless of why you're searching for sweet potato recipes, these selections are likely to include something you'll want to prepare and consume.

1. Poblanos and Sweet Potato on Black Bean Tostadas

You're going to start making these black bean tostadas as your go-to simple vegetarian meal. With heart-healthy ingredients like cabbage, black beans, sweet potatoes, peppers, and fresh herbs, it can be prepared in about 35 minutes. The crema brings everything together, and you can top it with crumbled cotija cheese for even more richness.

2. Sweet potato-based vegetarian chili cooked slowly

If you are unable to add meat to your vegetarian chili, add a lot of vegetables, such as tomatoes, bell peppers, red onions, and sweet potatoes. Two types of beans complete the dish, adding interest and body. This sweet potato chili may be enjoyed as a main course for your next tailgate or as a weekday meal.

3. Black bean and Zucchini Filled Sweet Potatoes

Here, cooking sweet potatoes in the microwave cuts down on cooking time, so in only 20 minutes, you can serve this high-fiber dinner. The black bean filling is combined on the burner while the potato cooks.

Top each potato with a wedge of lime and white cheddar cheese right before serving. Remember to store any leftovers as the veggie-bean mixture tastes delicious when topped on nachos or tucked into tacos.

4. Cheesecake with sweet potatoes and vanilla flavor

This delicious cheesecake has a graham cracker crust made with brown butter, enough cream cheese, and just the right amount of sweet potato. The outcome is a dessert that is both nostalgic and sophisticated, and the greatest part is that it only takes 20 minutes of actual work. Before removing the flesh and mashing the sweet potato, if you're in a hurry, microwave it.

5. Chile and molasses Sweet potatoes roasted

Though earthy molasses might seem a little too intense for sweet potatoes that have a hint of sweetness already, there's a whole new world of taste when you combine the thick, brown syrup with the sharpness of stone-ground mustard and the heat of jalapeño. The crisp-tender sweet potato wedges serve as a canvas for their delicious flavors.

6. Sweet potatoes loaded with kale and coconut

Sweet potatoes can be quickly cooked by popping them in the microwave. This step will cut your overall time by roughly thirty minutes, making this sweet potato dish ready in only thirty minutes. While the potatoes are cooking, the kale and chiles become delicate, and the inherent sweetness and earthy flavors of the potatoes are enhanced with a dash of citrus juice and ground allspice.

7. Pan Sheet Sweet potatoes and chicken

For busy cooks, sheet-pan dinners are the epitome of perfection. All of the ingredients for your meal—in this example, sweet potato wedges and chicken leg quarters—can be prepared simultaneously on the same dish. You'll save a ton of work, mess, and time by doing this. This dish is perfect for weeknights because it's really easy to prepare. You may swap out the greens (watercress for butter lettuce or any other green you have on hand) and herbs (sage is called for, but rosemary would also work).

8. Sweet potatoes baked in the oven

Sweet potatoes' inherent sweetness is enhanced when they are baked. Every time you use this traditional baked sweet potato recipe, the potatoes come out perfectly cooked. They can be eaten plain, straight out of the oven, or as a foundation for any number of toppings you choose.

9. Apple and Roasted Sweet Potato with Mustardy Kale Salad

This substantial salad for the main course is a nutritional powerhouse, loaded with fiber and protein. In a big bowl, mix the kale, roasted sweet potato, diced apple, and almonds. Drizzle with the tart mustard vinaigrette. After dressing, use clean hands to massage the kale to add some taste to the salad.

10. Buttermilk Pancakes with Sweet Potatoes

The addition of mashed sweet potatoes to pancake batter transforms ordinary pancakes into a delectably fluffy, delicate, and healthier option. The addition of cinnamon, nutmeg, and maple syrup to this batter gives the dish hints of warm caramel and vanilla. Buttermilk adds just the right amount of acidity to the pancakes.

11. Farro Bowl with a Vinaigrette of Pomegranates

This filling grain dish has salty feta, crisp fennel, caramelized sweet potato, and nutty farro. A pomegranate vinaigrette brings the whole dish together and elevates it to a whole new level. We promise you'll adore it!

12. Roasted Sweet Potatoes with Cheese

With two types of oozy cheese on top, these sweet potato wedges have the perfect balance of salty and sweet flavors. They only need four ingredients and cook in less than 30 minutes. They will probably be devoured so fast that you might want to double the recipe since they are that delicious.

13. Apple and Sweet Potato Soup with Walnuts and Cheese

This simple soup has a wonderful smoothness without even a hint of cream thanks to the richness of sweet potatoes and soft onions. This traditional fall supper pairs well with crisp apples and a side of tangy blue cheese. Nutmeg enhances the sweetness of the cooked sweet potato and apple.

14.Sweet potatoes stuffed with chickpeas

Do you need to eat extra protein? Make these vegetarian sweet potatoes with packed chickpeas and a dollop of seasoned yogurt on top.

The flavor of the chickpeas comes from a combination of cumin and spicy cinnamon, along with flat-leaf parsley and chives, though you can use other herbs if you want. Tarragon, dill, and basil also work well.

15.Maple-Sweet Potato Puree

The finest sweeteners for sweet potatoes are those with a rich flavor, such as maple syrup, molasses, or honey. Granted, brown sugar or even plain sugar works just as well, but the earthy tones of the potatoes bring out the distinct flavors of these all-natural sweeteners.

For this puree, ground nutmeg adds an extra flavor boost in the form of maple syrup. Even though sour cream is typically used in white potato purees, it offers a unique creaminess and richness that comes from dairy.

16. Corn salsa served with sweet potato and bean burritos

These burritos are loaded with fresh tomato-corn salsa, beans, lots of cheese, and crispy-tender shoestring sweet potatoes. Peel and then grate the potatoes, then bake and add to the tortilla filling. Please feel free to freeze any leftovers by wrapping the burritos in parchment paper.

Before wrapping up the ingredients, make sure everything has cooled completely to avoid the burritos becoming mushy.

17. Quinoa with Pesto, Kale, and Sweet Potatoes

Protein is abundant in this vegetarian sweet potato dish because of the fiber-rich quinoa and diced sweet potatoes, which provide a staggering 14 grams per serving. Two grams of protein are found in one cup of the mildly sweet potato. In addition, this dish's ingredients are all packed full of vitamins and minerals.

18. Sweet potatoes and chickpeas with roast chicken

Dinner in three simple steps: Arrange ingredients in piles on a sheet pan. Grill. Consume. In the oven, the potatoes get tender, the chicken cooks and the chickpeas become crispy. All of this is combined with a sprinkle of store-bought pesto to create a supper that takes about 20 minutes to prepare.

19. Coconut-Sweet Potato Casserole

Treat your family to this take on the traditional holiday side dish if they like sweet potato casserole and are willing to try something new. The brown sugar, pecan, and shredded coconut toppings are rich variations on the traditional Thanksgiving dish. Since there probably won't be any leftovers, get your scoop first.

20. Slow-Cooker Barbecue Sweet Potato Cooks

Bring out your reliable slow cooker and make these baked potatoes with it. Topped with cheddar cheese, barbecue sauce, sour cream, and rotisserie chicken—a great time-saver—each slow-baked potato dish. Is there anything not to love?

21. Sweet Potato Pie

There are two groups of people who enjoy holiday desserts: those who have never had sweet potato pie and those who can't imagine having Thanksgiving dinner without it. They will then be converted once they do. A sprinkling of powdered sugar or a dollop of whipped cream might not even register as a difference for some folks.

22. Chili with Smoked Turkey

Serve a large party with this smokey chili, which gets its flavor from poblano peppers, tomatillos, and even a dash of cinnamon, which are typical Mexican ingredients. A combination of beans, corn, and sweet potatoes complete this nutritious and cozy meal. Store any leftovers in the freezer and thaw them out for your next game day lunch.

23. Sweet Potato Latkes Served with Balsamic Vinegar and Brie Cheese

Whether it's a Tuesday in July or Hanukkah, fried potato latkes are always a good idea. But the use of sweet potatoes and the rich addition of creamy brie cheese make this dish unique. The latkes have a stark contrast from the balsamic vinegar drizzle, but the flavors work well together to create a tasty supper or side dish.

24. Bulgur and Roasted Sweet Potato Salad

Roasted sweet potatoes, sturdy bulgur, peppery watercress, salty feta, crisp pistachios, and pungent onion are all featured in this easy salad dish. First, bake the sweet potatoes after coating them with cumin; next, simmer the bulgur and whisk it together with a little vinegar and olive oil. After the entire grain has cooked, put the salad together and enjoy.

25. Rice with Sweet Potatoes

This hearty risotto is a vegetable-packed take on the traditional rice dish, made with rice and sweet potatoes. Don't worry if the only thing you know about risotto is that it requires continual stirring.

This recipe doesn't need to be watched over all the time, even if stirring is involved. Even though the entire dish just takes 40 minutes to prepare, it looks good enough to present to guests.

26. Gruyère and Sweet Potato Turnovers

Tender sweet potato, softened onions, and silky, wilted Swiss chard should be stuffed into flaky crusts. Bake with sharp Gruyère cheese for a hearty, exciting, and hands-on meal that's perfect for cold nights. Serve this dish with a hardy grain, such as barley or quinoa, and a green side salad to round it out.

27. Sweet potatoes with maple flavor and spicy pecan praline

Try this recipe if you can't decide between savory and sweet. After coating sweet potato wedges in a buttery maple glaze flavored with pepper, candied pecans flecked with lime and cayenne are added. This meal is a no-brainer for

Thanksgiving, but it also makes a classy side dish for a dinner party.

28.Sweet and Smoky Potato Burgers

While store-bought pre-made vegetarian burgers are readily available, preparing your meatless patties is also surprisingly simple. The base of this recipe is made up of sweet potato, beans, oats, and chia; a small amount of chipotle chile is added to offer a ton of smokey flavor. You can prepare these simple burgers in advance and freeze them for those evenings when you're stuck for ideas for dinner.

29.Brie and Sweet Potato Flatbread

This flatbread is an easy way to sate your appetite for pizza while sneaking in some veggies, whether it's served as an appetizer or as a main meal (served with a side salad). Brie is used in place of mozzarella in this recipe to create an incredibly creamy topping. This could easily become a go-to option for game nights, book groups, or any time you need a simple yet impressive dish because it's so easy to make—everything cooks at once in the oven.

30. Kale and Sweet Potato Tortilla Soup

Nutritious sweet potato and kale are combined with crunchy corn tortilla strips to create this delicately flavored tortilla soup. Serve as a vegetarian dish or add some protein by stirring in some shredded rotisserie chicken. Top it all off with radishes, avocado, and cilantro.

31. Sweet potatoes boiled

Sometimes a straightforward cooking technique brings out a vegetable's inherent deliciousness. This is what happens when you boil sweet potatoes. It's up to you whether to remove the skin or leave it on. In either case, you'll have soft sweet potatoes that are wonderful on their own or in other recipes.

32. Roasted Sweet Potatoes Served with Black Bean and Chipotle Chili

For this vegetarian chili and dinner, using canned black beans cuts down on cooking time.

While the sweet potatoes are roasting in the oven, make the chili. Add as many toppings as you like on top, such as avocado, cotija cheese, sour cream, and cilantro.

33.Leek and Sweet Potato Soup with Cream

Sweet potatoes, chicken broth, and sautéed leeks (cooked in bacon fat) are combined in this rich and creamy soup dish. Thickened with heavy cream, the soup takes on a luxurious texture. For a flavorful and cozy dinner, sprinkle some crispy bacon and chives on top before serving.

34.Latkes made with sweet potatoes

Grated sweet potatoes and russet potatoes are combined to give this latke recipe a distinct flavor and consistency. Make sure to squeeze out as much liquid as you can from the potato mixture for a crispier texture. Serve as a tasty snack or appetizer with seasoned herb sour cream.

35. Sweet Potato and Salmon Frittata

Although frittatas make a great morning or brunch dish, there's no denying that they taste just as well for dinner. Salmon and fresh sweet potatoes make for a flavorful and filling combo in this frittata. You'll adore how simple this dish is, and it only takes an hour to put together.

36. Potatoes with a Garlicky Herb-Butter Layer

This tasty side dish of potatoes is easy to prepare and has a crispy top and a creamy interior thanks to the combination of Yugon Gold and sweet potatoes. Although it requires some time to put together, it's quite simple and well worth the effort.

To ensure consistent layers, buy potatoes that are comparable in size and shape.

37. Quinoa with Sweet Potatoes, Kale, and Mushrooms

This vegetarian dish, which is full of healthy kale, quinoa, mushrooms, and sweet potatoes, is excellent on its own or as a side dish for chicken or salmon. With only thirty minutes of preparation time, it's ideal for a weekday supper. For a vegan take on this meal, omit the white wine and Parmesan cheese.

38. Soup with Winter Lentils

This vegetarian soup, loaded with lentils and veggies high in fiber, boils quickly and easily in one pot. This dish is great any night of the week, but it's especially good on a cold night since sweet potatoes give it an earthy sweetness.

39. Lentil Soup with Sausage and Mustard Greens

Lentils add a nutritious dose of veggies and nutrients to this hearty stew, along with sweet potatoes and mustard greens. To lessen the bitterness of the mustard greens, try cooking them with lentils and sweet potatoes. After that, savor the broth with a wonderful piece of crusty bread.

40. Pancakes with vegetables and sesame-fried eggs

Sweet potatoes give traditional veggie pancakes a delicious boost in this Korean-inspired recipe. Sweet potatoes shine in this delicious dish when combined with umami-rich cremini mushrooms and peppery scallions in a light batter. A sesame-fried egg cooked over easy is placed on top of everything, allowing the creamy yolk to mingle with the pancake for the ideal bite.

CHAPTER 4
POTENTIAL SIDE EFFECTS AND INTERACTIONS

May be ineffective in

- Treating cancer: It doesn't seem that eating potatoes can stop cancer deaths.
- Rectal and colon cancer. It doesn't seem that eating potatoes can prevent rectal or colon cancer.
- Heart attack. It doesn't seem like eating potatoes can stop heart attacks.
- Demise due to whatever reason. It doesn't seem that eating potatoes can stop death from any cause.
- Stroke. It doesn't seem that eating potatoes can prevent strokes.

Not Enough Data to Support Heart Disease. Eating purple potatoes appears to alleviate artery stiffness but not other heart disease risk factors, according to preliminary studies. Furthermore, eating potatoes does not reduce heart disease, according to population research.

Gastric distress (dyspepsia). According to preliminary studies, some people may find that drinking potato juice helps to relieve their gastrointestinal symptoms.

High blood pressure. Eating little purple potatoes may lower blood pressure slightly, according to preliminary studies.

Boils.

Burns.

Infections.

Being overweight.

arthritis of the bones.

Additional circumstances.

Adverse Reactions

When consumed by mouth: Eating ripe, spotless potatoes is Probably Safe. Taking pure, ripe potatoes, potato juice, or potato extracts as medication is POSSIBLY SAFE. Consuming fried potatoes may result in weight gain. Heartburn, bloating, and diarrhea can all result from consuming potato juice.

Eating sprouts, green potatoes, and potatoes with damage is Probably Not Safe. These may include toxic substances that cooking cannot get rid of. Sweating, headaches, flushing, nausea, vomiting, diarrhea, stomach discomfort, thirst, restlessness, and even death are among the symptoms that these toxic compounds can induce.

Potatoes when applied topically may not be safe, and there is insufficient and unreliable information available to determine any potential negative effects.

Particular Care and Cautions

When consumed by mouth: Eating ripe, spotless potatoes is Probably Safe. Taking pure, ripe potatoes, potato juice, or potato extracts as medication is POSSIBLY SAFE. Consuming fried potatoes may result in weight gain. Heartburn, bloating, and diarrhea can all result from consuming potato juice.

Eating sprouts, green potatoes, and potatoes with damage is Probably Not Safe. These may include toxic substances that cooking cannot get rid of. Sweating, headaches, flushing, nausea, vomiting, diarrhea, stomach discomfort, thirst, restlessness, and even death are among the symptoms that these toxic compounds can induce.

When rubbed upon the skin: Insufficient and unreliable information exists to determine the safety of potatoes or their potential side effects. Breastfeeding during pregnancy: Eating perfectly ripe potatoes while pregnant or nursing is LIKELY SAFE. However, insufficient trustworthy data is available to determine the safety of higher dosages used as medication. Be cautious and follow meal recommendations.

RELATIONSHIPS

Moderate Communication: Use caution when combining this mixture.

Thrombolytic drugs, which are medications used to dissolve blood clots, interact with POTATO

There is a substance in potatoes that prevents blood coagulation. Consuming high quantities of potatoes along with blood clot-dissolving medicines may make bleeding and bruises more likely.

Alteplase (Activase), anistreplase (Eminase), reteplase (Retavase), streptokinase (Streptase), and urokinase (Abbokinase) are a few drugs that are used to dissolve blood clots.

POTATO and succinylcholine interact

One drug that is occasionally administered during surgery is succinylcholine. The duration of succinylcholine may be prolonged if potatoes are consumed the night before surgery. This could make recovery from surgery more difficult.

Dosage

The right amount of potato depends on several variables, including the user's age, health, and other circumstances. There isn't enough scientific data available right now to establish a suitable range of dosages for potatoes. Keep in mind that natural products aren't always safe and that dosages are important. Before using, be sure to read the product labels carefully and speak with your doctor, pharmacist, or other healthcare provider.